Diseases, Diagnosis and Treatment

Volume 12:
The Hematological System

(Erythrocytes, Lymphocytes and Thrombocytes)

Solomon Barroa, R.N

Copyright 2013

All rights reserved. No part of this book may be reproduced by any means, electronic, mechanical, photocopying, recording, scanning or otherwise without permission from the author. The author reserves the right not to be responsible for the correctness, completeness or quality of the information provided. Liability claims regarding damage caused by the use of any information provided, including any kind of information that is incomplete or incorrect, will be rejected. The information contained in this book does not constitute medical advice, and is for information and educational purposes only. Consult your health care provider regarding health concerns.

To Dr. Lee Robbins, Mary Ann, Rosario, Vicente, Benedicto, and Robert.

Introduction and Purpose

Healthcare is an activity essential to all of us-that recieves greatly increased emphasis during periods of illness. People who practice healthcare, those who aid people in need are called healthcare professionals. Healthcare professionals require academic certification and licensure through extensicve study and diligent effort.

Choosing this career requires the integration of cognitive, affective and psychomotor skills. Healthcare professionals are devoted to ensuring quality care for all recipients of healthcare. Extensive training is needed to prepare physicians, nurses, medical assistants, physical therapists, radiology technicians, laboratory technicians and many more occupations to handle the wide range of diseases and disorders that afflict children and adults. Acquiring and refreshing extensive familiarity with diseases, diagnostic procedures and treatments is essential in order to provide the best care to our clients.

The volumes in this series and this particular book contain medical information that provides reference for healthcare professionals. Each volume presents a brief overview of anatomy and physiology, discussions about the pathophysiology of diseases with their common diagnostic procedures and treatment, a glossary with pronunciation guide, and quizzes/tests are located at the end of the book to assist the users of this text. The reader is advised that medical information change from time to time due to research and technological advancement. Healthcare is dynamic in all aspects.

Though it contains medical terminologies designed to provide review for healthcare professionals, a person without professional medical background is equally encouraged to read and learn from these medical discussions. The truth is that we and our loved ones will each at times be a recipient of healthcare. The descriptions of body systems, diagnoses and medical terminologies will be encountered dueing the process of caring for our own health and that of our loved ones. Some understanding of the nature of our bodies, of diseases that afflict us and of alternative treatment possibilities is very valuable for interacting effectively with our healthcare providers. Understanding each other will allow the process to be more effective for both providers and recipients.

The author encourages the reader to post reviews, comments and questions to:

solomon_barroa@yahoo.com

and the link :

http://www.amazon.com/Solomon-Barroa-R.N./e/B00AV3V34S/ref=sr_ntt_srch_lnk_1?qid=1361890980&sr=1-1

Thank you for buying this book in our series of volumes on systems of the body, their nature, illnesses, diagnoses and treatments. My deep intention is for the contents of these books to provide valuable information and satisfaction and help guide us to enhance health.

Table Of Contents

Chapter 1 Overview of Anatomy and Physiology of the Hematological System — 6

Chapter 2 Diagnoses and Treatment of the Diseases/Disorders affecting the Hematological System — 8

Anemia — *8*
Deep Vein Thrombophlebitis (DVT) — *9*
Hemochromatosis — *9*
Hemophilia — *10*
Malaria — *10*
Polycythemia Vera — *10*
Von Willebrand's Disease — *11*
Glossary — *12*
Anatomy of the Hematological System — *12*
The Types of Blood Cells — *12*
The Types of Leukocytes — *12*
Pathological Conditions of the Hematological System — *13*
Procedures and Treatment — *14*

Test 1 — 15
Test 2 — 18

Answer Key — 21

References — 25

Index — 26

Chapter 1 Overview of Anatomy and Physiology of the Hematological System

The hematological system is composed of cells such as RBC (red blood cell), WBC (white blood cell) and platelets. RBC is also known as erythrocyte. WBC is composed of agranulocytes, granulocytes and leukocytes. Agranulocytes are white blood cells with one large nucleus. They are composed of lymphocytes and monocytes. Lymphocyte is a type of white blood cell with a large dark stainable nucleus. Lymphocytes produce antibodies. Monocytes are formed in the bone marrow. They become macrophages after leaving the blood and function for phagocytosis. Granulocytes are white blood cells with multiple granules. They are composed of basophils, eosinophils and neutrophils. Basophils are characterized by large and dark granules. Eosinophils have a dense and reddish granule. Neutrophils have a neutral staining granule. They are produced in the bone marrow and functions for phagocytosis. Leukocytes are another type of white blood cells that fight infectious agents. A platelet cell is also known as thrombocyte.

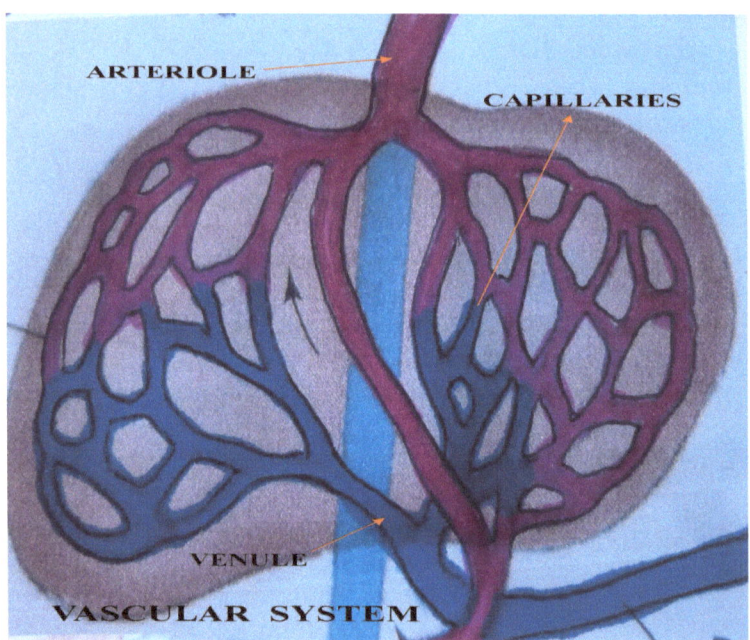

The blood is a liquid medium from which all chemical substances are transported throughout the body including foreign agents such as bacteria and parasites. It carries waste products such as urea and ammonia towards the kidney to be eliminated and carries nutrients from the intestines to the cells of the different organs of the body. The nutrients that the blood carries are albumin (protein), glucose (carbohydrate) and lipids (fats). Through the blood, gases such as oxygen maintain the perfusion of all the different systems in the body. Electrolytes such as sodium and potassium are also transported, eliminated and reabsorbed.

There are four blood types. These are types A, B, AB and O. These blood types contain different antigens and antibodies. An antigen is a foreign entity that triggers the production of antibodies. These antibodies are protein substances that neutralize an antigen.

In the process of blood transfusion, a mismatch between blood types will trigger an antibody and antigen reaction. This reaction results in agglutination or the clumping of a recipient's blood. It produces an acute hemolytic reaction through the destruction of erythrocytes. Symptoms such as fever, chills, chest pain, shortness of breath and sudden drops in blood pressure occur. The initial intervention will be to immediately stop the transfusion.

The blood type AB is considered a universal receiver because it can receive blood from all other blood types. This blood type cannot donate to blood types A and B because of its antigens. Blood type O is known as the universal donor because it can be donated to all blood types but can only receive blood of its own type. The blood type B can receive blood from types B and O but can only donate to types AB and B. Blood type A can receive blood from types A and O but can only donate to types AB and A.

The formation of a blood clot is important when there is a wound because it promotes healing and formation of a new skin. It is a process that stops the loss of blood from a damaged blood vessel. Blood clotting is also known as coagulation or thrombogenesis. This process is complex and requires different substances and chemical reactions. Initially the circulating platelets react to bind with collagen through glycoprotein receptors. Adhesion is started through this process. Blood factors for clotting such as the von Willebrand factor, are then released to further strengthen the adhesion. Calcium will be released in the platelets through the chemical changes brought about by the clotting factors. From these, the prothrombinase enzyme will be released. It converts prothrombin protein to an enzyme called thrombin. The enzyme thrombin will then convert the protein fibrinogen to fibrin. Finally fibrin forms the threads of clots.

Chapter 2 Diagnoses and Treatment of the Diseases/Disorders affecting the Hematological System

Anemia

This is a condition where there is a decrease in the number of red blood cells that are circulating in the body. Red blood cells provide oxygen to the body through its hemoglobin component. Hemoglobin is the protein inside the red blood cells that carries oxygen. The process of respiration enables the entry of oxygen into the red blood cells. The common causes of anemia are blood loss, impaired production or increased destruction of red blood cells.

There are different types of anemia; aplastic, hemolytic, pernicious, folic acid deficiency, sickle cell and iron deficiency. Aplastic anemia is due to impairment of the bone marrow's ability to produce an adequate supply of red blood cells. Hemolytic anemia is the premature destruction of red blood cells. Pernicious anemia is due to a deficient intrinsic factor that is needed in the absorption of vitamin B 12. Cobalamin (Vitamin B 12) is an essential component in the development of red blood cells.

Folic acid deficiency anemia is due to a deficiency in the intake of folic acid needed in the production of red blood cells. Sickle cell anemia is an inherited disorder where the red blood cells assume an abnormal rigid and sickle shape that obstructs blood flow and oxygenation. Iron deficiency anemia is due to insufficient dietary intake of iron needed for the association of hemoglobin inside the red blood cell.

The typical symptoms of anemia are fatigue, weakness, malaise and poor concentration. Pallor, palpitations, bounding pulse and chest pain may occur. Black and tarry stools occur in iron deficiency anemia. Jaundice and dark urine occurs in hemolytic anemia. Bleeding and bruising easily occurs in aplastic anemia.

Diagnosis of anemia requires differing diagnostic methods according to the type of anemia. The Schilling test is used to diagnose pernicious anemia. It involves using radioactive Vitamin B 12 to measure the amount of absorption in the body. Blood test for the protein ferritin is done to determine iron deficiency anemia. Bone marrow biopsy is performed to diagnose aplastic anemia. A sickle solubility test is done to diagnose sickle cell anemia. This test is done through acquiring blood films from a solution added to red blood cells.

Pernicious anemia is treated with lifetime intramuscular injections of Vitamin B 12. Iron deficiency anemia is treated with iron supplements. Hemolytic anemia can be treated with the removal of the spleen and corticosteroids if the cause is autoimmune disorder. Folic acid deficiency anemia is treated with folic acid supplements. Bone marrow transplants may be performed to treat aplastic anemia. Blood transfusion may be needed for managing sickle cell anemia.

Deep Vein Thrombophlebitis (DVT)

This is a condition where there is inflammation of the vein in the lower extremities in response to a thrombus (blood clot).
It is caused by clotting disorders and immobility such as sitting in an airplane for long period of time. The signs and symptoms of DVT in the affected leg are edema of the ankle and foot, warmth redness and cyanosis. It is usually asymptomatic in most cases.

Diagnosis is done through physical examination, doppler ultrasound, arteriography and blood coagulation studies. Venography is a procedure where a contrast media is injected into the affected vein to produce x-rays. Blood coagulation studies are series of blood tests that measures the ability of the blood to clot.

The treatment of DVT consists of medication such as anticoagulants, thrombolytics, analgesics, NSAID and antibiotics (if there is infection).
Anticoagulants are drugs that prevent blood clotting such as warfarin and heparin. Thrombolytics are drugs that dissolve existing clots such as streptokinase. Non-medical management involves elevation of the feet to reduce swelling and application of moist heat to reduce inflammation. Surgical removal, tripping and bypassing of the affected vein may be performed in some cases. The complication of DVT is pulmonary embolism.

Hemochromatosis

This is a condition where there is overload or excessive accumulation of iron in the body. The most common affected parts of the body are liver, pancreas, heart and testes. Hemochromatosis is caused by defective genes, chronic hemolysis (destruction of red blood cells), frequent blood transfusions and excessive iron supplementation. The most common symptom is a bronze grayish skin discoloration. Joint pain, drowsiness, weakness, shortness of breath, arrhythmia (irregular heartbeat), ankle edema (swelling of the ankle), polyuria (excessive urination), polydipsia (excessive thirst), abdominal swelling and pain also occur. Most of the symptoms manifested are due to the destruction of the organs involved.

Diagnosis is done with blood tests to measure the levels of iron in the blood. CT scan and MRI will be ordered also to determine the status of organs that are affected. Treatment consist of periodic phlebotomy (withdrawal of blood) to reduce the level of iron in the blood. Phlebotomy is done once a week until an acceptable level of iron in the blood is achieved.

Hemophilia

This is a condition where there is an absence of clotting factor. It is genetically inherited. There are 2 types of hemophilia; A and B. Hemophilia A is a deficiency in clotting factor 8 while Hemophilia B is a deficiency in clotting factor 9. The symptoms are frequent and extensive bruising, prolonged and spontaneous bleeding and hematuria. Headache, paralysis and coma may occur if there is bleeding in the brain. Swelling, tenderness and pain in the joints occur if there is bleeding in the joints.

Diagnosis is done with blood tests to measure the clotting time and blood levels of factor 8 and 9. There is no cure for hemophilia. Treatment involves infusion of the missing blood clotting factor that will stop the bleeding. The intake of warfarin, heparin, aspirin, ibuprofen are prohibited because these drugs prolong bleeding.

Malaria

This is a condition where there is infestation by the parasite plasmodia. It is transmitted by the bite of a female anopheles mosquito. There are 4 types of Plasmodium parasite; P. falciparum, P. malariae, P. ovale and P. vivax. The parasite travels to the liver and multiplies. Eventually it enters the blood stream and destroys the eryhtrocytes (red blood cells).
The destruction of RBC gives rise to symptoms such as high fever, chills, arthralgia (joint pain), muscle aches, headache, rapid shallow breathing, profuse perspiration, nausea and vomiting. The symptoms recur after a symptom free period.

Diagnosis is made through the microscopic analysis of the blood sample to confirm presence of the parasite. Severe cases of malaria are treated with chloroquine to kill the parasite. If the parasite is resistant, quinine and quinidine will be used. The drug primaquine is also administered to kill parasites in the liver and prevent recurrent attacks. Malaria can be prevented by avoiding the bites of infected mosquitos by using mosquito nets in bed, insect repellants, window screens, wearing long sleeves and staying indoors between dusk and dawn or at times when mosquitos become active.

Polycythemia Vera

This is a condition where there is overproduction of RBC from the bone marrow. The common symptoms are pruritus (itching), spleenomegaly (enlarged spleen), tinnitus (ringing in the ear), fatigue, diplopia (double vision), frequent headaches, nosebleeds, easy bruising and night sweats.

Diagnosis is done primarily with blood tests. Treatment involves phlebotomy (blood letting) to remove excess RBC and reduce viscosity of the blood. Interferon and hydroxyurea may be prescribed to reduce WBC. Antihistamines are also utilized to treat pruritus.

Von Willebrand's Disease

This is a condition where there is an absence of the Von Willebrand clotting factor. Just like hemophilia, this disease is also inherited. The symptoms are easy bruising, frequent nosebleeds, heavy bleeding from cuts, hematuria and swollen painful joints.

Diagnosis involves blood test to determine the missing clot factor. Treatment is done with the infusion of the missing factor during a bleeding episode. Desmopressin is also administered to stimulate release of the missing clot factor.

Glossary

Anatomy of the Hematological System

The Types of Blood Cells

Agranulocytes (ai-gran-u-lo-saits) = are white blood cells with one large nucleus. They are composed lymphocytes and monocytes.

Erythrocyte (e-rith-ro-sait) = is a red blood cell.

Granulocytes (gran-u-lo-saits) = are white blood cells with multiple granules. They are comprosed of basophils, eosinophils and neutrophils.

Leukocyte (loo-ko-sait) = is a white blood cell.

Thrombocyte (throm-bo-sait) = is a platelet cell.

The Types of Leukocytes

Basophil (ba-so-fil) = a type of white blood cell with large and dark granules.

Eosinophil (e-o-sin-o-fil) = is a type of white blood cell with dense and reddish granules.

Lymphocyte (lim-fo-sait) = is a type of white blood cell with large dark staining nucleus. Lymphocytes produce antibodies.

Monocyte (mon-o-sait) = is a type of white blood cell that is formed in the bone marrow. It becomes a macrophage after leaving the blood. It functions for phagocytosis.

Neutrophil (nu-tro-fil) = is a type of white blood cell with neutral staining granules. It is produced in the bone marrow and functions for phagocytosis.

Pathological Conditions of the Hematological System

Acute lymphocytic leukemia (a-kyut lim-fo-si-tik loo-ke-me-a) = is a condition where malignant immature lymphocytes predominate in the bone marrow and the bloodstream.

Acute myelogenous leukemia (a-kyut mai-e-loj-e-nus loo-ke-me-a) = is a condition where malignant immature granulocytes predominate in the bone marrow and the blood stream.

Aplastic anemia (a-plas-tik a-ne-me-a) = is a condition where there is a failure of the production of blood cells due to a defect in the development of bone marrow cells.

Chronic lymphocytic leukemia (kro-nik lim-fo-si-tik loo-ke-me-a) = is a condition where malignant mature lymphocytes predominate in the bone marrow and lymph nodes. It progresses slowly.

Chronic myelogenous leukemia (kro-nik mai-e-loj-e-nous loo-ke-me-a) = is a condition where both the malignant mature and immature granulocytes are present in the blood stream. It is a progressive and long term disease.

Dyscrasia (dis-krae-ze-a) = is a condition where there is an abnormal composition or disorder of the cellular elements in the blood.

Erythrocytopenia (e-rith-ro-sai-to-pe-ne-a) = is a condition where there is a deficiency in the number of red blood cells.

Granulocytopenia (gran-u-lo-sai-to-pe-ne-a) = is a condition where there is a low concentration of granulocytes in the blood resulting in a decreased resistance to infection.

Hemolytic anemia (he-mo-li-tik a-ne-me-a) = is a condition where the number of red blood cells are greatly reduced due to its destruction.

Hemoglobinopathy (he-mo-glo-bin-op-a-the) = is a condition where there is a genetic defect in the creation of a hemoglobin structure.

Hemophilia (he-mo-fil-e-a) = is a condition where there is excessive bleeding due to a congenital defect and absence of factor VIII for blood clotting.

Leukocytopenia (loo-ko-sai-to-pe-ne-a) = is a condition where there is a decrease in the number of white blood cells in the blood.

Multiple myeloma (mul-ti-pl mai-e-lo-ma) = is a condition where there is a malignant cancer of the bone marrow. It is a progressive tumor of cells that produce antibodies that eventually invades the bone marrow destroying the bone structure.

Pernicious anemia (per-nish-us a-ne-me-a) = is a condition where there is a deficient number of matured erythrocytes due to the body's inability to absorb vitamin B 12.

Polycythemia vera (pol-e-sai-the-me-a ver-a) = is a condition where there is an excessive volume of red blood cells.

Purpura (pur-pu-ra) = is a condition where there are numerous pinpoint hemorrhages and collection of blood under the skin. It produces a red purple discoloration on the skin.

Sickle cell anemia (sikl sel a-ne-me-a) = is a disease where a genetic blood disorder creates a rigid and sickle shaped red blood cell. The sickling of the cell results in the occlusion of the blood vessels and ischemia thereafter.

Thalassemia (thal-a-se-me-a) = is an inherited condition where there is a defective ability in producing hemoglobin.

Procedures and Treatment

Blood transfusion (blud trans-fu-zhun) = is a procedure of transfusing a whole blood that is taken from a donor. Proper matching and screening is done prior to the transfusion.

Bone marrow biopsy (bon ma-ro bai-op-se) = is a procedure of introducing a needle to the bone marrow cavity and aspirating samples for purposes of diagnosing a condition.

Bone marrow transplant (bon mar-ro trans-plant) = is a procedure where the bone marrow cells from a donor are infused to a recipient with leukemia and other blood conditions.

Erythrocyte sedimentation rate (e-rith-ro-sayt sed-e-men-tae-shun raet) = is a procedure where venous blood is collected and an anticoagulant is added to detect the rate or speed at which the erythrocytes settles out of plasma.

Partial thromboplastin time (par-shul throm-bo-plas-tin taim) = is a procedure that measures the presence of factors that act in the early phase of the coagulation process.

Prothrombin time (pro-throm-bin taim) = is a procedure that measures the elapsed time from the addition of calcium to a plasma sample and the appearance of a clot. In general, it is a test to measure the ability of the blood to clot.

Test 1

I. Matching type.
Match selection A with selection B with the appropriate word/s. There could be one or more answer/s from the selection.

Selection A

_____ 1. Blood type AB
_____ 2. Blood type
_____ 3. Blood type B
_____ 4. Blood type A

Selection B

a. universal donor
b. donates to AB & B
c. universal recipient
d. cannot donate to A & B
e. donates to AB & A
f. receives from A & O
g. receives from B & O

II. Multiple Choice. Choose the appropriate word/s to complete the following statements. There could be one or more answer/s from the selection.

1. (a. Agranulocytes b. Lymphocytes c. Monocytes d. Granulocytes) are white blood cells with one large nucleus. It composes lymphocytes and monocytes.

2. (a. Erythrocyte b. Hemoglobin c. Hematocrit d. Thrombocyte) is a red blood cell.

3. (a. Agranulocytes b. Granulocytes c. Monocyte d. Lymphocyte) are white blood cells with multiple granules. They are composed of basophils, eosinophils and neutrophils.

4. (a. Thrombocyte b. Leukocyte c. Erythrocyte d. Hematocrit) is a white blood cell.

5. (a. Leukocyte b. Hematocrit c. Erythrocyte d. Thrombocyte) is a platelet cell.

6. (a. Basophil b. Monocyte c. Lymphocyte d. Eosinophil) is a type of white blood cell with large and dark granules.

7. (a. Basophil b. Monocyte c. Eosinophil d. Lymphocyte) is a type of white blood cell with dense and reddish granules.

8. (a. Monocyte b. Basophil c. Lymphocyte d. Neutrophil) is a type of white blood cell with large dark staining nucleus. It produces antibodies.

9. (a. Neutrophil b. Basophil c. Lymphocyte d. Monocyte) is a type of white blood cell that is formed in the bone marrow. It becomes a macrophage after leaving the blood. It functions for phagocytosis.

10. (a. Neutrophil b. Basophil c. Eosinophil d. Monocyte) = is a type of white blood cell with neutral staining granules. It is produced in the bone marrow and functions for phagocytosis.

III. Identification Identify the terminologies that are defined in the following statements.

1. _____ = is a condition where malignant immature lymphocytes predominate in the bone marrow and the bloodstream.

2. _____ = is a condition where malignant immature granulocytes predominate in the bone marrow and the blood stream.

3. _____ = is a condition where there is a failure of the production of blood cells due to a defect in the development of bone marrow cells.

4. _____ = is a condition where malignant mature lymphocytes predominate in the bone marrow and lymph nodes. It occurs in slow progression.

5. _____ = is a condition where both the malignant mature and immature granulocytes are present in the blood stream. It is a progressive and long term disease.

6. _____ = is a condition where there is an abnormal composition or disorder of the cellular elements in the blood.

7. _____ = is a condition where there is a deficiency in the number of red blood cells.

8. _____ = is a condition where there is a low concentration of granulocytes in the blood resulting in a decreased resistance to infection.

9. _____ = is a condition where the number of red blood cells are greatly reduced due to its destruction.

10. _____ = is a condition where there is a genetic defect in the creation of a hemoglobin structure.

11. _____ = is a condition where there is excessive bleeding due to a congenital defect and absence of factor VIII for blood clotting.

12. _____ = is a condition where there is a decrease in the number of white blood cells in the blood.

13. _____ = is a condition where there is a malignant cancer of the bone marrow. It is a progressive tumor of cells producing antibodies that eventually invade the bone marrow destroying the bone structure.

14. _____ = is a condition where there is a deficient number of matured erythrocytes due to the body's inability to absorb vitamin B 12.

15. _____ = is a condition where there is an excessive volume of red blood cells.

16. _____ = is a condition where there are numerous pinpoint hemorrhages and collection of blood under the skin. It produces a red purple discoloration on the skin.

17. _____ = is a disease where a genetic blood disorder creates a rigid and sickle shaped red blood cell. The sickling results in the occlusion of the blood vessels and ischemia thereafter.

18. _____ = is an inherited condition where there is a defective ability in producing hemoglobin.

19. _____ = is a procedure of transfusing whole blood that is taken from a donor. Proper matching and screening is done prior to the transfusion.

20. _____ = is a procedure of introducing a needle to the bone marrow cavity and aspirating samples for the purpose of diagnosing a condition.

21. _____ = is a procedure where the bone marrow cells from a donor are infused to a recipient with leukemia and other blood conditions.

22. _____ = it is a procedure where venous blood is collected and an anticoagulant is added to detect the rate or speed at which the erythrocytes settles out of plasma.

23. _____ = is a procedure or a test that measures the presence of factors that act in the early phases of the coagulation process.

24. _____ = is a procedure or a test that measures the elapsed time from the addition of calcium to a plasma sample and the appearance of a clot. In general, it is a test to measure the ability of the blood to clot.

Test 2

1. An impairment of the bone marrow's ability to produce red blood cell is a characteristic of (a.aplastic anemia b.hemolytic anemia c.pernicious anemia d.bone marrow cancer e.none of the above).

2. A deficiency in intrinsic factor occurs in (a.aplastic anemia b.pernicious anemia c.sickle cell anemia d.iron deficiency anemia e.none of the above).

3-4. The (a.vitamin B 12 b.cobalamin c.A & D d.none of the above) is an essential component in the development of red blood cells to prevent (a.aplastic anemia b.pernicious anemia c.sickle cell anemia d.iron deficiency anemia e.none of the above).

5. The occurrence of sickle cell anemia involves (a.blood flow obstruction b.decrease tissue oxygenation c.genetic anomaly d.all of the above e.none of the above).

6. The symptoms of anemia may include (a.easy bruising b.jaundice c.all of the above d.none of the above).

7. Easy bruising does not occur in aplastic anemia (a.true b.false c.none of the above d.maybe).

8. Schilling's test is a diagnostic test for (a.aplastic anemia b.pernicious anemia c.sickle cell anemia d.iron deficiency anemia e.none of the above).

9. Jaundice does not occur in hemolytic anemia (a.true b.false c.none of the above d.maybe).

10. The protein ferritin in the blood is tested to determine (a.aplastic anemia b.pernicious anemia c.sickle cell anemia d.iron deficiency anemia e.none of the above).

11. Radioactive vitamin B 12 is utilized in Schilling's test (a.true b.false c.none of the above d.maybe).

12. Aplastic anemia is treated with (a.immunosupressant drugs b.anticoagulants c.bone marrow transplantation d.none of the above).

13. Sickle cell anemia is managed with (a.antibiotic b.anticoagulants c.blood transfusion d.none of the above).

14. Spleenectomy is performed to treat hemolytic anemia (a.true b.false c.none of the above d.maybe).

15. DVT (deep vein thrombophlebitis) involves (a.thrombus b.lower extremities c.inflammation d.all of the above e.none of the above).

16. Sitting in an airplane for a long period of time does not cause DVT (a.true b.false c.none of the d.maybe).

17. In general, the symptoms of DVT include (a.ankle edema b.cyanosis c.asymptomatic d.all of the above e.none of the above).

18. Diagnostic tests for DVT include (a.venography b.arteriography c.blood coagulation studies d.all of the above e.none of the above).

19. Untreated DVT leads to (a.pulmonary embolism b.congestive heart failure c.kidney failure d.none of the above).

20. The treatment of DVT consist of (a.tripping b.bypassing c.removal d.all of the above e.none of the above).

21. An excessive accumulation of iron in the body is called (a.hemolytic anemia b.spleenic disorder c.hemochromatosis d.none of the above).

22-23. Hemophilia B is a deficiency in clotting factor (a.7 b.9 c.6 d.8) and hemophilia A is a deficiency in clotting factor (a.7 b.9 c.6 d.8).

24. The symptoms of hemophilia may include (a.arthritis b.paralysis c.all of the above d.none of the above).

25. The common symptom of hemochromatosis is (a.bronze grayish skin color b.polyuria c.arrhythmia d.none of the above).

26. Arrhythmia may occur in hemochromatosis. (a.true b.false c.none of the above d.maybe).

27. Hemophilia is treated with (a.warfarin b.heparin c.all of the above d.none of the above).

28. Malaria involves (a.bite of a mosquito b.plasmodium parasite c.communicable disease d.none of the above).

29. Phlebotomy is done once a week in hemochromatosis (a.true b.false c.none of the above d.maybe).

30. The destruction of RBC (red blood cells) in malaria gives rise to symptoms such as (a.arthralgia b.chills c.vomiting d.all of the above e.none of the above).

31. Resistant plasmodium parasite in malaria are killed with (a.chloroquine b.doxycycline c.quinidine d.none of the above).

32. The drug (a.chloroquine b.primaquine c.doxycycline d.quinidine e.none of the above) is used in malaria treatment to prevent recurrent attacks).

33. PV (Polycythemia vera) involves (a.overproduction of RBC from the bone marrow b.acummulation of RBC in the spleen c.excessive number of RBC in the blood vessel d.none of the above).

34. The symptoms of PV are (a.pruritus b.spleenomegaly c.diplopia d.all of the above).

35. Interferon maybe prescribed in PV (a.true b.false c.none of the above d.maybe).

36. Hydroxyurea is never prescribed in PV (a.true b.false c.none of the above d.maybe).

37. VW (Von Willebrand's) disease involves (a.absence of clotting factor b.systemic infection c.autoimmune disorder d.none of the above).

38. The symptoms of VW include (a.arthritis b.hematuria c.all of the above d.none of the above).

39. Frequent nosebleeds occur in VW (a.true b.false c.none of the above d.maybe).

40. Drug such as (a.aspirin b.warfarin c.desmopressin d.none of the above) is prescribed to stimulate release of missing clot factor in VW.

Answer Key

Test 1

I. Matching type. Match column A with column B. There could be one or more answer/s from the selection.

C, D 1. Blood type AB
A 2. Blood type O
B, G 3. Blood type B
E, F 4. Blood type A

Blood type AB is a universal receiver. This blood type cannot donate to blood types A and B because of its antigens. Blood type O is known as the universal donor because it can be donated to all blood types but can only receive its own blood type. Blood type B can receive blood from types B and O but can only donate to types AB and B. Finally blood type A can receive blood from types A and O but can only donate to types AB and A.

II. Multiple Choice Choose the appropriate word/s to complete the following statements. There could be one or more answer/s from the selection.

ABC 1. Agranulocytes (ai-gran-u-lo-saits) are white blood cells with one large nucleus. They comprise the lymphocytes and monocytes.

A 2. Erythrocyte (e-rith-ro-sait) is a red blood cell.

B 3. Granulocytes (gran-u-lo-saits) are white blood cells with multiple granules. They form the basophils, eosinophils and neutrophils.

B 4. Leukocyte (loo-ko-sait) is a white blood cell.

D 5. Thrombocyte (throm-bo-sait) is a platelet cell.

A 6. Basophil (ba-so-fil) is a type of white blood cell with large and dark granules.

C 7. Eosinophil (e-o-sin-o-fil) is a type of white blood cell with dense and reddish granules.

C 8. Lymphocyte (lim-fo-sait) is a type of white blood cell with large dark staining nucleus. These cells produce antibodies.

D 9. Monocyte (mon-o-sait) is a type of white blood cell that is formed in the bone marrow. It becomes a macrophage after leaving the blood. It functions for phagocytosis.

A 10. Neutrophil (nu-tro-fil) is a type of white blood cell with neutral staining granules. It is produced in the bone marrow and functions for phagocytosis.

III. Identification Identify the terminologies that are defined in the following statements.

1. Acute lymphocytic leukemia (a-kyut lim-fo-si-tik loo-ke-me-a) is a condition where malignant immature lymphocytes predominate in the bone marrow and the bloodstream.

2. Acute myelogenous leukemia (a-kyut mai-e-loj-e-nus loo-ke-me-a) is a condition where malignant immature granulocytes predominate in the bone marrow and the blood stream.

3. Aplastic anemia (a-plas-tik a-ne-me-a) is a condition where there is a failure of the production of blood cells due to a defect in the development of bone marrow cells.

4. Chronic lymphocytic leukemia (kro-nik lim-fo-si-tik loo-ke-me-a) is a condition where malignant mature lymphocytes predominate in the bone marrow and lymph nodes. It is a progressive and long term disease.

5. Chronic myelogenous leukemia (kro-nik mai-e-loj-e-nous loo-ke-me-a) is a condition where both malignant mature and immature granulocytes are present in the blood stream. It is a progressive and long term disease.

6. Dyscrasia (dis-krae-ze-a) is a condition where there is an abnormal composition or disorder of the cellular elements in the blood.

7. Erythrocytopenia (e-rith-ro-sai-to-pe-ne-a) is a condition where there is a deficiency in the number of red blood cells.

8. Granulocytopenia (gran-u-lo-sai-to-pe-ne-a) is a condition where there is a low concentration of granulocytes in the blood resulting in a decreased resistance to infection.

9. Hemolytic anemia (he-mo-li-tik a-ne-me-a) is a condition where red cells are destroyed resulting in the number of red blood cells becoming greatly decreased.

10. Hemoglobinopathy (he-mo-glo-bin-op-a-the) is a condition where there is a genetic defect in the creation of a hemoglobin structure.

11. Hemophilia (he-mo-fil-e-a) is a condition where there is excessive bleeding due to a congenital defect and the absence of factor VIII for blood clotting.

12. Leukocytopenia (loo-ko-sai-to-pe-ne-a) is a condition where there is a decrease in the number of white blood cells in the blood.

13. Multiple myeloma (mul-ti-pl mai-e-lo-ma) is a condition where there is a malignant cancer of the bone marrow. It is a progressive tumor of cells that produce antibodies that eventually invades the bone marrow destroying the bone structure.

14. Pernicious anemia (per-nish-us a-ne-me-a) is a condition where there is deficient number of matured erythrocytes due to the body's inability to absorb vitamin B 12.

15. Polycythemia vera (pol-e-sai-the-me-a ver-a) is a condition where there is an excessive volume of red blood cells.

16. Purpura (pur-pu-ra) is a condition where there are numerous pinpoint hemorrhages and collections of blood under the skin. It produces a red purple discoloration on the skin.

17. Sickle cell anemia (sikl sel a-ne-me-a) is a disease in which a genetic blood disorder creates a rigid and sickle shaped red blood cell. The sickling results in the occlusion of the blood vessels and ischemia follows thereafter.

18. Thalassemia (thal-a-se-me-a) is an inherited condition in which there is defective ability to produce hemoglobin.

19. Blood transfusion (blud trans-fu-zhun) is a procedure of transfusing whole blood that is taken from a donor. Proper matching and screening is done prior to the transfusion.

20. Bone marrow biopsy (bon ma-ro bai-op-se) is a procedure of introducing a needle into the bone marrow cavity and aspirating samples for the purpose of diagnosing a condition.

21. Bone marrow transplant (bon mar-ro trans-plant) is a procedure where bone marrow cells from a donor are infused into a recipient who has leukemia or other blood conditions.

22. Erythrocyte sedimentation rate (e-rith-ro-sayt sed-e-men-tae-shun raet) refers to a procedure where venous blood is collected and an anticoagulant is added to detect the rate or speed at which the erythrocytes settles out of plasma.

23. Partial thromboplastin time (par-shul throm-bo-plas-tin taim) is a procedure or a test that measures the presence of factors that act in the early phase of the coagulation process.

24. Prothrombin time (pro-throm-bin taim) is a procedure or a test that measures the elapsed time from the addition of calcium to a plasma sample and the appearance of a clot. In general, it is a test to measure the ability of the blood to clot.

Test 2

1. A
2. B
3. C
4. B
5. D
6. C
7. B
8. B
9. B
0. D
11. A
12. C
13. C
14. A
15. D
16. B
17. D
18. D
19. A
20. D
21. C
22. B
23. D
24. C
25. A
26. A
27. D
28. B
29. A
30. D
31. C
32. B
33. A
34. D
35. A
36. B
37. A
38. C
39. A
40. C

References

I would like to express my gratitude to:

Dr. Lee Robbins for his support in writing this book.

Anatomy and Physiology, Wiley and Sons, New Jersey, 2007
Fundamentals of Nursing 7th Edition, Mosby, Canada, 2009
Gerontological Nursing 2nd Edition, ANCC, Maryland, 2009
Medical – Surgical Nursing 4th Edition, Prentice Hall, New Jersey, 2008
NCLEX PN, Saunders, Missouri, 2003
NCLEX RN, Mosby, Missouri, 1999
Nursing Assistants, Mosby, Philadelphia, 2004
Nursing Interventions and Clinical Skills, Mosby, Missouri, 2004
Nursing Procedures and Protocols, Lippincott, Philadelphia 2003
Pathophysiology of Disease 2nd Edition, Appleton and Lange, 1997
Pharmacology in Nursing 21st Edition, Mosby, Missouri 2001
Principles and Practice of Psychiatric Nursing 6th edition, Mosby, Missouri 1998
The Johns Hopkins Consumer Guide to Medical Tests, Medletter Associates Inc, New York, 2001
The Johns Hopkins White Papers, Hypertension and Stroke, Medletter Associates Inc, New York, 2003
Wikipidea Free Internet Dictionary

Index

Acute lymphocytic leukemia, 13, 22
Acute myelogenous leukemia, 13, 22
Agranulocytes, 6, 12, 15, 21
ankle edema, 9, 19
antibiotics, 9
antigen, 7
Aplastic anemia, 8, 13, 18, 22
arrhythmia, 9, 19
arthralgia, 10, 19
autoimmune disorder, 8, 20
Basophil, 12, 15, 16, 21
bleeding, 10, 11, 13, 17, 22
blood, 6, 7, 8, 9, 10, 11, 12, 13, 14, 15, 16, 17, 18, 19, 20, 21, 22, 23
Blood transfusion, 9, 14, 23
blood vessels, 14, 17, 23
bone marrow, 6, 8, 10, 12, 13, 14, 16, 17, 18, 20, 22, 23
Bone marrow biopsy, 8, 14, 23
Bone marrow transplant, 14, 23
bruising, 8, 10, 11, 18
chloroquine, 10, 20
Chronic lymphocytic leukemia, 13, 22
Chronic myelogenous leukemia, 13, 22
cyanosis, 9, 19
Deep Vein Thrombophlebitis (DVT), 9
Desmopressin, 11
diplopia, 10, 20
drowsiness, 9
Dyscrasia, 13, 22
Eosinophil, 12, 15, 16, 21
eryhtrocytes, 10
Erythrocyte, 12, 14, 15, 21, 23
Erythrocytopenia, 13, 22
factor VIII, 13, 17, 22
fatigue, 8, 10
female anopheles mosquito, 10
fever, 7, 10
fibrin, 7
Folic acid deficiency anemia, 8
glycoprotein, 7
Granulocytes, 6, 12, 15, 21
Granulocytopenia, 13, 22
hematuria, 10, 11, 20
Hemochromatosis, 9
hemoglobin, 8, 13, 14, 16, 17, 22, 23
Hemoglobinopathy, 13, 22
hemolysis, 9
Hemolytic anemia, 8, 13, 22
hemolytic reaction, 7
Hemophilia, 10, 13, 19, 22
heparin, 9, 10, 19
hydroxyurea, 10
Interferon, 10, 20
iron, 8, 9, 18, 19
Iron deficiency anemia, 8
Leukocyte, 12, 15, 21
leukocytes, 6
Leukocytopenia, 13, 22
Lymphocyte, 6, 12, 15, 16, 21
Malaria, 10, 19
Monocyte, 12, 15, 16, 22
Multiple myeloma, 13, 23
muscle aches, 10
nausea, 10
Neutrophil, 12, 16, 22
nosebleeds, 10, 11, 20
Partial thromboplastin time, 14, 23
Pernicious anemia, 8, 14, 23
phagocytosis, 6, 12, 16, 22
phlebotomy, 9, 10
Plasmodium parasite, 10
platelet, 6, 12, 15, 21
Polycythemia vera, 14, 20, 23
polydipsia, 9
polyuria, 9, 19
primaquine, 10, 20
prothrombin, 7
Prothrombin time, 14, 23
prothrombinase, 7
pruritus, 10, 20
Purpura, 14, 23
quinidine, 10, 20
quinine, 10

rapid shallow breathing, 10
red blood cells, 8, 9, 10, 13, 14, 16, 17, 18, 19, 22, 23
Sickle cell anemia, 8, 14, 18, 23
sickle solubility test, 8
spleenomegaly, 10, 20
Thalassemia, 14, 23
thrombin, 7
Thrombocyte, 12, 15, 21
Thrombolytics, 9
thrombus, 9, 19
tinnitus, 10
universal donor, 7, 15, 21
universal receiver, 7, 21
Venography, 9
viscosity, 10
Von Willebrand, 11, 20
warfarin, 9, 10, 19, 20
weakness, 8, 9
Willebrand factor, 7

***Kindly write a review about this book to help other readers that could benefit from this text. Thank you.

And please feel free to browse my other books @ Amazon.com

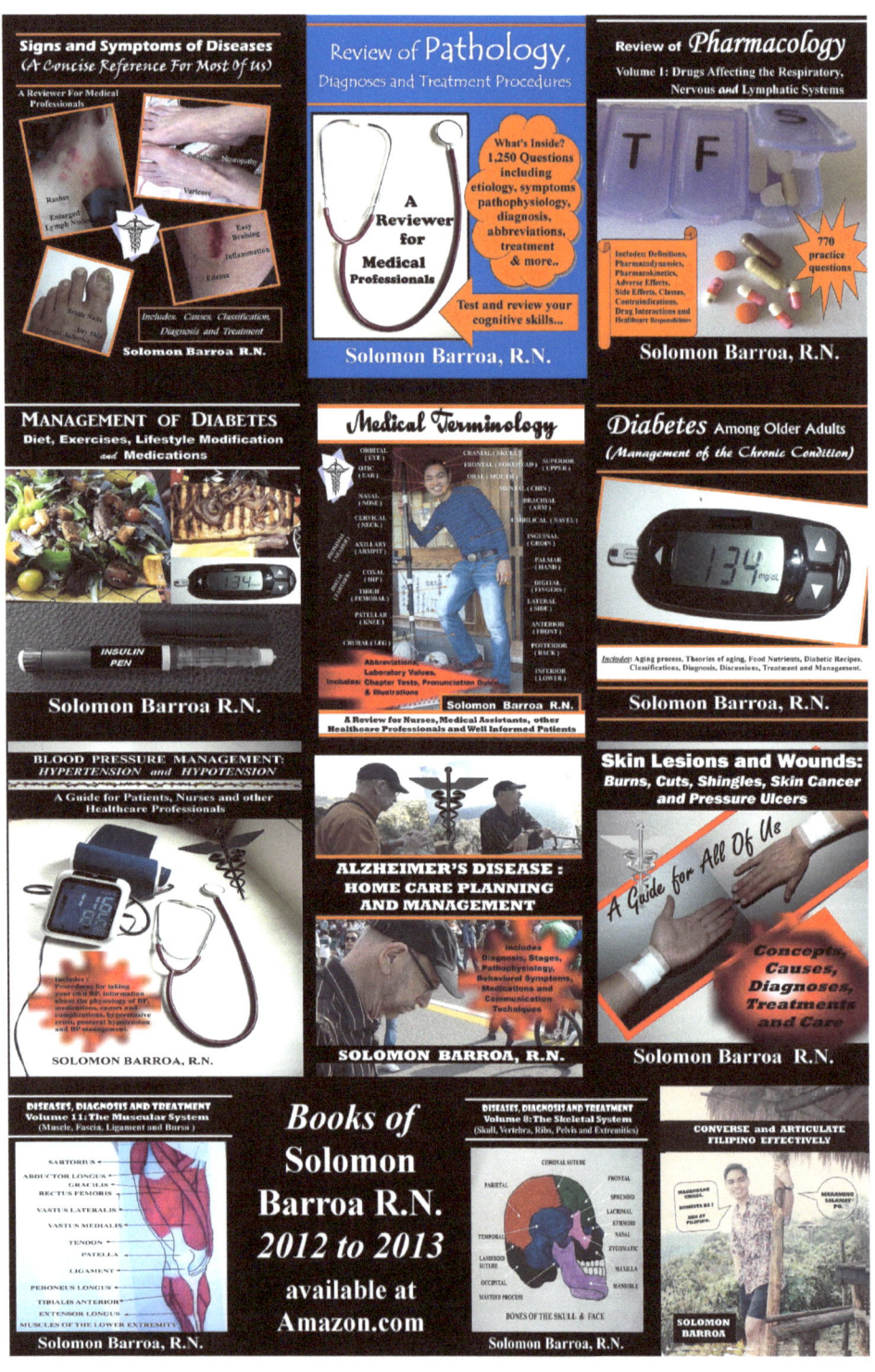

Connect with me online :

Facebook: http://www.facebook.com/solomon.barroa
Twitter: https://twitter.com/solomonbarroa
Amazon: amazon.com/author/solomonbarroa
LinkedIn: http://www.linkedin.com/in/solomonbarroa

www.ingramcontent.com/pod-product-compliance
Lightning Source LLC
Chambersburg PA
CBHW050426180526
45159CB00005B/2423